Essential Oils

How to Use Essential Oils to Ease Hormonal Imbalances, Anxiety, Stress and Restore Health and Beauty to your Life

I0449806

Introduction

I want to thank you and congratulate you for downloading the book, *"Essential Oils"*.

This book contains proven steps and strategies on how to use essential oils to treat depression, mood swings, stress and to improve your skin health among other things.

As a woman, when your hormones are in balance, you can live a physically and physiologically healthy life. However, when hormonal imbalances occur, they lead to problems such as vaginal dryness, lower libido, infertility, hot flashes, irregular menses, mood swings, depression, irritability, and sleep disturbances. Because of hormonal imbalances, some women occasionally gain or lose weight, while others cannot lose weight even if they eat healthy and exercise.

It is important to understand that your endocrine system, the system that controls hormones is very sensitive to stress, anxiety, or depression caused by lack of sleep, chronic pain, toxins, inflammation, too much work, and eating processed or genetically modified foods.

Once under extreme stress, levels of cortisol rise, which causes a drop in sex hormones such as estrogen and progesterone. A reduced level of these hormones triggers problems such as weight gain, irregular menses, infertility, and estrogen dominance.

Other problems emanating from hormonal imbalances include breast tenderness, hypothyroidism, hair loss, and increased storage of belly fat. Hormonal imbalances as you can clearly see have adverse negative effects.

Unfortunately, when most women experience a hormonal imbalance, their first instinct is a change of diet and lifestyle habits in a bid to offset hormonal issues. While this is indeed an effective way to balance your hormones, completely changing your diet is not always sustainable and a change of diet is not always effective.

What then is the most effective way to balance the hormones, feel beautiful and energetic, and reduce anxiety? The answer is two words: essential oils. This book will open your eyes to the world of possibilities with essential oils. We shall look at the most effective essential oils for women, and outline how to use these oils to achieve optimum health, beauty, vigor, energy, ease anxiety, and many other uses that are beneficial to your overall wellbeing.

Thanks again for downloading this book, I hope you enjoy it!

this book are for clarifying purposes only and are the owned by the owners themselves, not affiliated with this document.

Table of Contents

Conclusion

Essential Oils and Women's Health

If you deal with a lot of stress emanating from a hectic work or home schedule, your hormones are often under constant imbalance. As earlier outlined in this guide, hormonal imbalances are bad for you. Even though you are a busy mom/daughter/career woman, who always feels 24HRS is not enough to accomplish all you may desire or set out to accomplish at the start of a new day (which often leads to stress and anxiety that causes hormonal imbalances), you do not need to worry. Stress is a daily part of the life bestowed upon us.

However, to live a healthy and fulfilled life, you need to find ways to offset the stress of everyday life, and which causes negative hormonal imbalances in your body. This is where essential oils come in to help you achieve relaxation, gain more energy and vigor to accomplish more, feel beautiful, relaxed, and stress free. So, what exactly are essential oils?

Essential oils are concentrated liquids made from various parts of plants such as roots, stems, flowers, bark, and other materials. These plants' extracts posses healing properties that make them efficient at protecting your body, boosting immunity, and healing common ailments such as migraines.

Essential oils are antiseptic, anti-bacterial, anti-fungal, antioxidants and antiviral in nature, which makes them very useful to your overall health and well-being. Essential oils are applicable topically, inhaled, diffused, or orally as single products or as blends with other oils. For internal application, you should take proper care because oils are highly concentrated products that can cause problems.

Although essential oils are not hormone rich, their rich properties trigger hormone synthesis and balance. When buying an essential oil product, be aware that not all essential oils are the same in quality and safety. Therefore, always buy oil brands certified as pure therapeutic grade and labeled as medicinal.

Before we look at various essential oils that you can use to deal with different problems, let us first look at how to use essential oils.

How to Use Essential Oils

There are different ways to use essential oils; these range from topical skin application, inhaling, and body massage, to soaking in a bath.

How you use an essential oil depends on the type of oil you are using and the intended results. This is because some oils are more effective when applied topically to specific areas of your body, while some work best when directly inhaled into the lungs.

Whichever method of application you choose, the oils should influence your hormonal balance because most have estrogenic properties called phytoestrogens that control secretion of hormones.

Be aware that a majority of essential oils are very strong and concentrated; therefore, you need to dilute them before directly applying to the hair or scalp. To dilute, add base oil, or dilute in the essential oil in herbal rinse or floral water. When making a blend, ensure the content of the essential oil is 1-3 percent and the rest is carrier oil. You may probably be wondering what carrier oils or base oils are; thus, let us look at that.

Carrier Oils

Carrier oils are oils added to essential oils to dilute them mainly because using concentrated essential oils can lead to skin irritation, or respiratory problems when inhaled.

As an adult woman, a 2-3 percent dilution with carrier oil is recommended, or a 1 percent during pregnancy. To dilute, add 1-2 drops of essential oil to 50 drops of carrier oils such as:

Coconut oil
Extra virgin olive
Sweet almond
Apricot kernel oil
Jojoba

Avocado oil

Essential Oil Application Methods

To use essential oils after diluting, adopt any of these application methods:

Inhalation

Rub 1-2 drops of essential oils such as lavender into your palms, cup your hands over your nose, and take about 4-6 deep breaths of the diffused oil scent. You can also add few drops of your preferred oil to a bowl of boiling water, put a towel over your head, and breathe into the steam for 5-10 minutes.

To make this method of application more effective, make various blends using various oils with a few drops of carrier oils like jojoba or almond oil.

Diffusion

Choose any essential oil or already made blends and add a number of drops into your diffuser according to the package directions. If using spearmint or peppermint essential oil, use in moderation because its aroma is very strong.

Cotton-ball or Diffusion

Place 1-3 drops of your favorite oil or blend onto a tissue or cotton ball, position it near your nose, and inhale. When doing the initial inhale, use 1 drop to check for sensitivity to the oil because a strong aroma may in some cases worsen a headache or migraine.

Aroma-Therapeutic Bath

Add 5-10 drops of essential oil or blend into a bathtub, preferably diluted in a tablespoon of a carrier if you have a sensitive skin. Avoid adding oils to running water because this will cause evaporation, which will reduce efficiency.

Cold Compress

This method of application works best for headaches and other pains that accompany the menstruation period. Add around 5 drops of your preferred essential oil or blend into 1-quart icy or very cool water. Soak a cloth or cotton ball into the bowl, and place it at the back of the neck or onto your forehead.

Topical Massage

Here, you can blend different oils. Mix your blend of carrier and essential oils in a bottle and then roll it between your hands to combine.

To use, apply 1-4 drops onto the fingers, gently massage the oils onto your forehead, and the back of the neck or the temples. Be careful not to touch the eyes.

How to Balance Your Hormones

As we have stated, different essential oils have varying effects on your body and overall wellbeing. In this section, we shall look at, and outline the various essential oils you can use to enhance hormonal balance within your body.

Let us begin our journey to perfect hormonal balance by looking at how to balance your adrenal glands

Adrenal Balance: How to Use Essential Oils to Balance Your Adrenal Glands

The adrenal glands regulate stress by balancing the production of the cortisol hormone. The function of the adrenal gland works best when you are sleeping or restful; stressful conditions can interrupt cortisol balance and thus, the function of the adrenal gland.

Adrenal imbalance manifests through symptoms such as:

*Brain fog
*Food cravings
*Inability to relax especially when under stress
*Hyperactivity at odd hours of the morning or at evening
*Fatigue after waking up

Essential oils that work best to balance the adrenal gland and production of cortisol include basil, lavender, and anise.

Basil Oil

This oil boosts your body's ability to fight physical and emotional stress, which helps you relax.

This finding draws its basis from a scientific research paper published in Evidence-Based Complementary and Alternative Medicine journal. In the study, scientists analyzed the effect of daily intake of basil extracts on women for a period of 6 weeks. 39% of the patients experiencing chronic stress experienced lesser stress symptoms, improved memory, better sleep, and lesser tiredness.

How to Use Basil Oil

Basil essential oil is especially suited to you if you experience chronic exhaustion, stress, and anxiety. To use basil oil, rub a few drops of quality basil essential oil on your forearms to bring balance to your adrenals. Apply some at the tragus- the ear's adrenal gland point located above your ear lobe. Apply the oil before you retire to bed because adrenal balance and sleep affect each other.

To enhance restful sleep, adapt lavender aromatherapy by creating a mist of water and lavender in a spray bottle and spray the mixture on your pillow. To make the oils work better, add in some anise essential oil.

Thyroid Dysfunction: How to Use Essential Oils to Optimize Your Thyroid Function

The thyroid hormone helps you control body temperature and metabolism. When your thyroid hormone is out of balance, it births issues such as insomnia, dry hair and skin, body temperature fluctuations, depression, and unmanageable weight loss or weight gain. Essential oils that can optimize thyroid regulation include myrtle, lemongrass, and licorice.

Myrtle Oil

This oil triggers the functionality of thyroid. A research study by Dr. Daniel Penoel found that myrtle oil has the potential to balance and restore hormonal balance in the ovaries and thyroid.

This volatile oil contains activate ingredients such as eugenol and elemol that are anti-microbial and soothing, and can work irrespective of whether the organs are under or over performing.

How to Use Myrtle Oil

To use the essential oil, rub a few drops of the oil on the big toe of your foot or at base of the foot. Locate the reflexology point of your thyroid at the fleshy area underneath the big toe.

You can also apply the oil at the thyroid area located below the base of the throat; i.e. the Adam's apple. To make the oil more effective, blend myrtle with lemongrass oil.

Licorice Oil

Licorice oil is a strong antidepressant that alleviates problems such as depression and fatigue. To use the oil, rub a drop of the oil onto your hands, rub your hands to warm it up, and then inhale the warm scent of licorice oil to boost your mood and feel better.

Essential Oils That Foster Ovary Balance

Did you know that your ovaries bear the task of producing helpful hormones such as progesterone and estrogen? These two hormones control processes like your menstruation and menopause. When there is an imbalance of these hormones, it can wreak havoc on your reproductive system.

Women with this imbalance can experience symptoms such as lower libido, irregular menses, infertility, PMS, problematic menopausal hot flashes, and sweats.

One way to correct hormonal imbalance is to adopt a simple liver detox because the liver controls the production of estrogen and other sex hormones.

Here is how you can do that:

Clary Sage Essential Oil

Clary Sage essential oil is effective at alleviating symptoms linked to progesterone and estrogen imbalances and for menstrual pains.

To use the oil, dilute 2-3 drops of the oil in almond oil and rub the blend on your ankles daily. If chronic pain accompanies your menstruation cramps, rub the mixture on the ovary and stomach area to relieve pain.

This oil also has components that alleviate pain, reduce stress, and balance hormones in your body. To enhance the effectiveness of Clary sage oil, add geranium essential oil to the blend. Add the blend of the two into a warm bath and soak for a few minutes.

How To use Essential oils to deal with PMS

Premenstrual syndrome occurs because of hormonal imbalances that occur prior to your menstruation cycle. To re-balance the hormones in your body, use the following essential oils and blends

PMS Bath Blend

In a warm bath, blend the following essential oils:

2 drops of lavender essential oil
2 drops of geranium
2 drops of chamomile
3 drops of Clary sage

Before adding the blend to your bath, add ¼ cup of Epsom salt to prevent the oils from floating on the water.

PMS Hormonal Balance Blend

1 drop of Ylang Ylang essential oil
1 drop of geranium oil essential oil
2 drops of Clary sage oil essential oil

Clary sage boosts the release of feel good dopamine in your brain and elevates your mood. The oil also helps monitor estrogen level in the body. Geranium facilitates the release of adrenal hormones and inhibits hormone fluctuations.

Menstrual Massage Blend

Create a perfect essential oil blend that you can rub on various areas such as your back, the abdomen, and your entire body.

3 drops of rose essential oil
3 drops of Clary sage essential oil
6 drops of lavender essential oil
4 teaspoons of a carrier oil of choice

For carrier oil, you can use oils such as jojoba, sweet almond, and coconut oil.

Essential Oils for Menstrual Cramps and Pains

As discussed earlier, you can use various essential oils to achieve different goals. One of these is alleviating menstrual pain and cramps. Here are the various essential oils you can use:

Clary Sage Essential Oil

Clary sage is an effective pain remedy because it produces a feeling of "narcotic like high" that works well for many women. Use it to reduce pain caused by menstrual cramps and as a tonic to your uterine lining.

The estrogenic properties present in Clary sage make it effective at regulating menstrual cycle. You can also use it to treat stress and anxiety. Avoid using the oil if you are pregnant, but you can use it during labor under the care of a skilled practitioner. You should not consume alcohol before, during, or after massaging or inhaling clary sage essential oil.

Chamomile Essential Oil

Chamomile essential oil has powerful antispasmodic properties that help relieve labor pains and menstrual cramps. You can use German or Roman chamomile.

Tea Tree Essential Oil

Tea tree oil stimulates the release of hormones and boosts circulation of blood in a bid to relief menstrual cramps. The oil also has strong antiseptic and antiviral properties that treat yeast infections, herpes, and cystitis.

In addition, the essential eliminates toxic substances that contribute to hormonal imbalances. Its sudorific properties help detox your body of harmful toxins that can lead to hormonal imbalance.

Peppermint Essential Oil

The main reason why peppermint oil is so effective is its ability to relieve headaches that occur before or during your menstrual cycle. The oil has the capacity to lower the intensity of headaches or migraines to the same extent as 1,000 mg of acetaminophen.

In addition, peppermint causes no adverse reactions, and can eliminate brain fog that occurs during ovulation.

Jasmine Essential oil

Jasmine oil has found uses in childbirth since ancient times. This oil is a potent uterine tonic that strengthens the tissues of your reproductive organs. Jasmine oil has parturient properties that help your reproductive organs contract during labor. Once rubbed on the abdomen, the oil can lower contraction pain and facilitates an easier labor.

Wintergreen Essential Oil

Wintergreen essential oil contains methyl salicylate, a sweet smelling substance that relieves strong pain such as the one synonymous with menstrual cramps.

Apply the oil directly on the muscle spasm or where there is pain including along the spine. Oils work best when used 2-4 times a day depending on the intensity of the pain.

Essential Oils for Libido and Fertility

Failure to conceive can be due to factors such as hormonal imbalance, stress, thyroid problems, and taking certain medications. Although infertility problems have many complex underlying causes, essential oils can ease many conception related problems.

A few of these oils can boost chances of conception and reduce mood problems that disrupt your hormones and in the process, negatively influence the overall wellness of your reproductive system.

Oils that work best here are calming oils that boost the functionality of your reproductive system. They include:

German Chamomile Essential Oil

Known to fight inflammation, this deep blue oil has an active ingredient referred to as azulene, which accounts for its effectiveness. The German version of chamomile calms the nerves, reduces depression and stress, and can be a good remedy against painful fibroids or cysts.

However, do not use chamomile when pregnant, particularly if you are prone to miscarriages. Additionally, if trying to conceive, it is advisable to use the essential oil before the beginning of your ovulation.

Geranium Essential Oil

This essential oil stimulates your adrenal cortex, which helps monitor or balance hormone secretion and functionality. Geranium also has the ability to detox your lymphatic system, and is an effective antidepressant suitable for instances when you are experiencing mood swings.

To use geranium essential oil, blend it with a few drops of yarrow essential oil. The oil works by preventing inflammation in your sexual organs and can relieve pelvic congestion. Yarrow can also improve your urinary system.

Rose Otto Essential Oil

Although expensive, Rose Otto essential oil effectively addresses PMS pain, controls your menses, and facilitates conception. The oil works by relaxing your uterus; its aphrodisiac properties make you feel confident of your sexuality.

Rose Otto also treats depression that can occur after you miscarry or a failed IVF. The oil also boosts your libido and can trigger the production of cervical mucus.

You should only use it before pregnancy and discontinue its use after conceiving.

Lavender Essential Oil

Well known to calm and relax a troubled mind, lavender calms you down and balances your endocrine system. The oil is part of the PregPrep's conception kit that is a blend between juniper, grapefruit, lemon oil, and lavender. If looking to conceive, consider adding lavender to your bath to achieve its therapeutic benefits.

Cinnamon Essential Oil

The oil from cinnamon plant is sweet, spicy, and warm; it calms your nerves, awakens your senses, and boosts circulation to reproductive organs. When well diluted, the cinnamon oil should boost sexual desire.

You can blend the oil with Clary Sage, which is a natural libido enhancer that controls estrogen levels and balances other sexual hormones. The sweet and warming patchouli oil is another blend worth a try. Patchouli oil treats vaginal yeast infections, boosts your libido, and enhances your endocrine glands.

Essential Oils for Stress and Insomnia

Stress is part of the life we all know. To live healthy and fulfilled lives, we have to learn how to manage stress in a healthy and holistic manner. As indicated earlier, essential oils are very effective at easing stress, insomnia, and anxiety.

To ease stress and sleep better, consider using these essential oils:

Clary Sage Essential Oil

Clary sage is a super oil prepared from mint botanical family and has properties that stimulate calmness and euphoria. It has a warm and mellow scent that relaxes and uplifts your mood, and thus effective at easing mood swings common during menses or postpartum depression that occurs after childbirth. The oil also has sedative properties that soothe your brain and combat insomnia symptoms.

A 2014 study discovered that the oil lowers cortisol levels by 36 percent and considerably boosts levels of the thyroid hormone. The study was conducted on 22 post-menopausal women with some previously diagnosed with depression. The study found that the oil lowered their stress levels and offered anti-depressant effect that improved mood and general wellbeing.

To use the oil to boost your mood, enhance relaxation, and better sleep, rub it at the bottom of your feet. You can also diffuse the oil and inhale it to reduce stress and improve your memory. However, if you suffer from fibroids, avoid long-term use of the oil.

Rosemary Essential Oil

Rosemary oil has a sharp scent capable of fighting stress and anxiety; it also improves memory and focus. The oil enhances your brainpower and accuracy levels especially when you are experiencing mood swings. Rosemary also fights fatigue, and boosts energy in women.

To boost your memory and focus during the day, topically massage rosemary oil on your palms each morning or alternatively add 2-3 drops into a bath. However, the recommendation is to inhale rosemary oil because this increases its effectiveness and is easy to do. Simply place 2 drops of diluted rosemary essential oil onto your palms and sniff it.

Sweet Marjoram Essential Oil

This oil improves blood circulation and eases menstrual cramps. The strong scent of the sweet oil relaxes your body and mind, treats related problems such as insomnia, and promotes deeper sleep. Sweet marjoram works best when blended with other oils such as chamomile, bergamot, and lavender.

To use the essential oil, place a blend of this oil onto your palms and inhale into it. Try carrying a little diluted oil in a cotton pad or scarf with you, or insert the cotton pad in your bra or breast pocket. The aroma from the oil will help you feel relaxed and energized throughout the entire day.

Ylang Ylang Essential Oil

Part of why Ylang Ylang effectively fights anxiety and improves concentration is because of the sedative effect it has on the brain. Ylang Ylang lowers the pulse rate and blood pressure, thus relieve symptoms of attention deficit disorders. The oil is most effective when inhaled to boost attentiveness or alertness, as well as to relieve stress and anxiety.

By inhaling its aroma, or topically applying it on the back, wrists, neck, or feet, you can improve blood circulation and heal hypertension. For topical applications, rub and press the mixture onto various points on your face and take care not to touch your eyes.

You can also dilute this essential oil in carrier oil such as extra virgin olive and add to hot water bath to fight stress and enhance concentration.

Blue Cypress Essential Oil

Premenstrual syndrome can cause symptoms such as stress, depression, headaches, and mood swings. Blue cypress oil relaxes and controls your breathing patterns to make you less anxious.

The easiest way to use this oil is by placing a few drops of the essential oil in your palms and inhale when you experience anxiety. A majority of users appreciate the pleasant scent blue cypress has to offer and apply it as scent trigger when dealing with challenging projects.

Try rubbing 1-2 drops of diluted blue cypress essential oil into your palms, cup them over the nose, and then take about 4-6 slow and deep breaths. Alternatively, place 2-4 drops of the oil onto a cotton ball, use a zip lock bag to secure it, and carry this with you.

To use the essential oil in milder concentration, pour boiling water into a dish, add in blue cypress oil, drape a towel over your head, and breathe into the steam. For this application, you can blend with other oils such as rosemary and eucalyptus essential oils.

Frankincense Essential Oil

This essential oil is useful in many ways including stress relief, and restoring hormonal balance when blended with other oils. Frankincense has elements such as Incensole Acetate, which lowers symptoms of stress and depression. It does this by activating the limbic system of the brain, and allows the brain to focus without disruption. The oil also carries oxygen required by your brain to stimulate the limbic area of the brain such as the hypothalamus, pituitary, and pineal glands.

The easiest way to use frankincense oil to fight anxiety is rubbing it on the feet to realize a calming effect, and to heal any anxiety and mood disorder. You can mix frankincense with other oils like peppermint and lavender to create blends.

You can use a diffuser to diffuse Frankincense oil to offer the most-needed nerve calming benefits especially during meditation and prayers.

How to Fight Insomnia: A Blend

To fight insomnia, combine these oils and then massage into the skin or add 2 teaspoons into your bath water.

4 ounces vegetable oil
2 drops ylang ylang oil
3 drops frankincense
10 drops sandalwood oil
10 drops lavender oil
15 drops bergamot oil

These oils are also effective when directly inhaled into your lungs. To use in a diffuser, omit the vegetable oil and then pour the mixture onto a simmering pan of water. Breathe into the fumes before going to bed. Use this until your sleeping patterns improves.

Essential Oils for Beauty and Hair

Because the world has a wide array of essential oils, it is impossible to run out of an essential oil option in any area of your life. As such, you can use essential oils to have flawless, magazine worthy skin or hair.

While any essential oil that fosters overall wellbeing will make you feel and look beautiful, below are essential oils suited for overall beauty inclusive of skin and hair.

Tea Tree Blend

Acne is a condition caused by overproduction of sebum, the oil that protects the skin, or hormonal imbalance caused by birth control pills.

You can blend tea tree oil with lavender to promote healthy skin and fight weary and damaged skin. The two oils are rich in antiseptic properties that help kill bacteria and other microorganisms.

To use, dilute 1 drop each of tea tree, lavender, geranium, or German chamomile with 50 drops carrier oil such as jojoba. Clean your face (or acne riddled spot) and apply diluted oil sparingly using a cotton pad every night until the acne disappears.

Lemon Essential Oil

Lemon oil is an effective treatment for dry and curly hair because it causes the oil glands to generate more oil that allows for healthier, stronger, and shiny hair. Lemon essential oil also treats dandruff especially if you apply it regularly.

Routinely using this essential oil should also destroy hair parasites such as lice and fleas. However, do not expose your hair to sunlight after using this oil because the oil can oxidize after exposure to the sun, which can affect your hair color.

Cedar-Wood Essential Oil

Cedar wood oil moisturizes your hair and treats a dry and oily scalp. The oil also stimulates the scalp and hair follicles. If you suffer from baldness, the essential oil can treat hair loss and dandruff. Further, cedar-wood is an antiseptic and an astringent, properties that protect the scalp and minimize bleeding caused by minor abrasions.

Ylang Ylang Essential Oil

Although it has a wide array of uses, Ylang Ylang oil is famous in tropical Asian cultures for its ability to enhance smooth skin and naturally healthy hair. The essential oil has potential to balance an oily scalp and restore optimum production of sebum.

Ylang Ylang oil is also a natural antiseptic and a tonic agent that heals an irritated scalp in addition to killing microorganism responsible for scalp infections. Ylang is also good at improving the flow of blood into the scalp and hair follicles to facilitate hair growth.

Bergamot Essential Oil

This oil is famous for its power to sooth the scalp, aid in hair growth, and gives your hair a natural shine.

To use it, blend the oil with coconut and castor oil to make a hair tonic. Adding a few drops of a hair conditioner can make it effective at boosting its smoothing power, as well as balancing the pH of your scalp.

Be aware that the oil might increase your photosensitivity after applying on your skin; therefore, to avoid possible skin burns, avoid going into the sun immediately after use.

Vetiver Essential Oil

This oil comes from the roots of khus grass. It prevents hair loss resulting from high body heat. This is because the oil has cooling properties that calms and soothes the entire body. Besides healing oily scalp and acne, this oil offers excellent relaxation benefits especially when used for massages or bath.

Lavender Essential Oil

Many users of lavender oil can attest to the fact that it restores balance of natural oils in the scalp, which leads to moisturized and dandruff-free hair. The oil is analgesic, antiseptic, and anti-inflammatory in nature, which makes it very efficient at treating a dry and flaky scalp.

Lavender essential oil also soothes and nourishes an itchy scalp, while still offering relief to an inflamed scalp. Regularly massaging this essential oil into your scalp should reduce hair loss and give you shiny and soft hair.

How to Use Essential Oils for Healthy Hair

To massage thin hair, keep the base oil in your blend as light as possible. To do so, dilute essential oils in base oils such jojoba oil, grape-seed, peach kernel, and apricot kernel.

If your hair is thick and coarse, use rich nourishing oils such as sesame, evening primrose, rose hip, hemp, olive, and avocado oils. Ensure you make a balanced hydrating agent by combining good quantities of essential and corresponding base oils. For instance, use 3-5 drops of an essential oil with a teaspoon or 5 ml of a base oil such as olive oil.

Once you have diluted an essential oil, massage it onto your hair and scalp, allow the blend to soak for 1 hour or overnight, wash with your usual shampoo, and allow the hair to dry.

Please note that essential oils normally evaporate quickly; thus, you should not leave them exposed for long.

Essential Oils for Optimum Digestion and Metabolism

Essential oils you can use for optimum digestive health and metabolism include:

Fennel Essential Oil

This oil comes from a plant of the parsley family. It balances the digestive and hormonal system. Women who have used fennel oil have reported improvement in digestive discomfort and constipation symptoms.

The best way to use the oil is to diffuse and inhale from a handkerchief or inhaler to solve digestive problems. However, do not use the oil during pregnancy or if you are suffering from epilepsy.

Lemon Essential Oil

The oil contains d-Limonene, vitamin C, and other minerals that fight intestinal parasites responsible for poor metabolism and weight gain. Lemon essential oil also helps the body eliminate toxins stored in fat cells.

You can use the essential oil in a number of ways such as inhalation, adding 1-2 drops in drinking water, and massaging the oil into cellulite areas to thin fat cells.

Grapefruit Essential Oil

This oil has an active ingredient referred to as d-limonene, which prevents bloating and helps the body break fatty acids into energy. Grapefruit oil also contains the antioxidant Lycopene, which cleanses the lymphatic system while detoxifying the body.

The easiest way to use this oil is to add 1-2 drops to a glass of drinking water daily preferably during breakfast to burn fat and flush out toxins.

Rosemary Essential Oil

Rosemary essential oil is effective as a gastrointestinal remedy because of its ability to calm muscles, cure bloat, and relieve constipation.

To relax, boost circulation, aid detox, and healthy digestion, combine 7-8 drops of rosemary oil with 7-8 drops fennel or geranium. Add the blend to 2 ounces of carrier oil such as jojoba or sweet almond and combine in a safe container to make a relieving massage oil.

Peppermint Essential Oil

This oil treats stomach upsets, indigestion, and inflammation in the GI tract, and boosts flow of bile. Peppermint oil also boosts level of gastric juices, relieves bloat and discomfort, as well as gas in the intestines.

To relieve stomach upsets that cause diarrhea, dilute 2 drops peppermint in 2-3 drops olive or coconut oil and rub onto the stomach. You can also add a drop of peppermint to drinking water to treat a sour stomach, or look for already made capsules.

Lavender Essential oil

This one is a powerhouse at easing flatulence, indigestion, and other mood swing symptoms that come with menopause. Lavender also reduces seasonal allergies and aids liver detoxification.

Conclusion

Using essential oils will not only help you feel healthier, younger, radiant, and beautiful, as this book has shown you, it will also help you manage a number of womanly conditions such as menstruation pain and cramps, acne-riddled skin and unhealthy hair, menopause related symptoms, as well as the many manageable conditions we have outlined here.

Thank you again for purchasing this book!

I hope this book has provided you with all the information you need to live a happy, healthier, and beautiful life. The rest is up to you; put what you have learned here into good use: you shall not regret it.

Finally, if you enjoyed this book, would you be kind enough to leave a review for this book on Amazon?

Thank you and good luck!

Melissa Keane

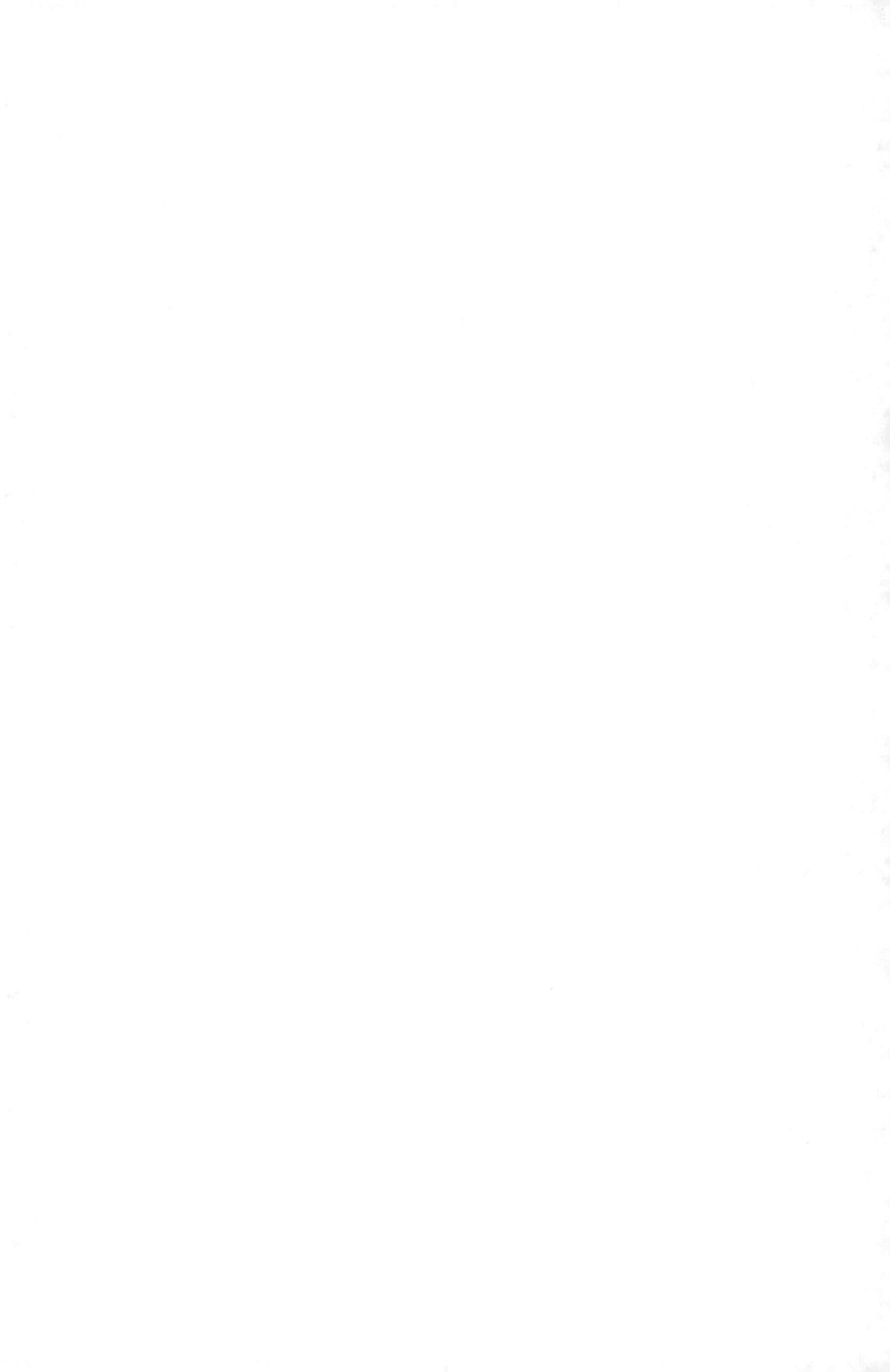

www.ingramcontent.com/pod-product-compliance
Lightning Source LLC
Chambersburg PA
CBHW062031280526
45787CB00005B/2283